Love Your Body, Change Your Life

Book 1:
Know Who You Are

EMMA WRIGHT

DEDICATION

For M and M. Love always.

CONTENTS

ACKNOWLEDGEMENTS   i

INTRODUCTION   Pg 1

1 UNDERSTAND YOU   Pg 17

2 THE CREATIVE SOUP   Pg 20

3 THE RESISTANCE   Pg 31

4 THE DIFFERENT ASPECTS OF "I"   Pg 35

5 YOUR POTENTIAL   Pg 46

6 MEDITATION   Pg 52

7 PERSONAL INVENTORY   Pg 61

8 TOOLKIT   Pg 71

9 'TIL WE MEET AGAIN   Pg 75

ACKNOWLEDGMENTS

I couldn't have chosen a creative career without my sister, who leads by example and inspires me to accomplish things that matter.

My brother and sister-in-law who make a living from their creativity and always see the best in people.

Thanks to my mothers, all four of you, in order of appearance: Mum, for passing on an expansive love of reading and for calling me a writer way before I could see it in myself; Faysie, for being the ears and wisdom I needed when life went wonky; Ellie, for being the role model I always wanted; Ann, for being a living example of unconditional love.

Dad for encouraging me to follow my heart, always, regardless of … anything.

My creative friends who inspired me and kept me real.

My mummy friends who kept me sane when the grenade that is children exploded into my life.

My long-time friends who lent an ear, gave a hug, or pulled out a stern sort-yourself-out when necessary.

A special thanks to Tom, who made me promise to keep going, and Suzie, who relentlessly demonstrates what following a dream requires.

Everyone else who touched my life, allowed me to create and grow and, of course, those of you who bought my work.

Caroline for editing that not only made my words sparkle, but brought heart, generosity, love, and guidance. Deeply humbled to have worked with you.

Thanks to all of you darling people who proofread, beta-read, gave me feedback: Karlie, Jo and Kim (to name a few). So lucky to have you in my court.

Last, but in no way least (in fact, most), my family: My immediate one, G (I'm so proud of the life we are creating) and our two darlings (seriously, love like I've never known); and my wider scrambling messy fabulous whanau (Maori for extended family, including blood relatives and extra close friends); you know who you are.

Lastly to my readers. Without you none of this would have been possible. Stay blessed.

X

.

INTRODUCTION TO THE SERIES

How It Begins

Darkness cannot drive out darkness;
only light can do that.
Hate cannot drown out hate;
only love can do that.

~ Martin Luther King

When I was nineteen, I told my parents I was bulimic. They didn't believe me. Or, at least they didn't believe it was really a problem.

I was so "together" on the outside. They saw my eating disorder as a kind of blip, phase, or thing I was trying out like a new fashion, or type of music.

What they failed to see was the bottomless self-hatred I kept veiled from the world. I desperately wanted to be the sparkly person my parents thought I was. So I slipped back into the jail of my secret and kept trying to fix myself – to change what was wrong with me, to tame my body so I could like myself and have a better life.

It took twenty-five years to escape that jail. It took that long to accept myself, love myself, and find the freedom and peace I sought.

I've written this series of books as a possible way out from the sentence that food and weight obsession can impose on day-to-day life. I had full-blown bulimic hell. You may have the same, or something different: A constant disappointment in your body; a nagging sense of doing the same thing again and again, hoping you'll get a different result; the fear of eating what you really want; a wild out-of-control feeling; a lifetime of dieting; obesity. All of these can come from the same place and, as you will see, can be healed in the same way.

Almost every day, it seems, another weight loss or healthy eating program becomes available. I used to be compelled by each new offering. Buoyed up, I'd think, this will be the ticket. This time will be different. I'll find the strength to commit to what they say. I'll start tomorrow, and it will all work out.

But it never quite did. Nothing lasted. Nothing parked up and changed me the way I really wanted.

And worse still, trying to solve the issues of my body— through good nutrition and exercise, plus other things like understanding emotions, setting up habits, looking to past events, making commitments—all gave some temporary relief but, in the end, only worked to deepen my despair. With every failure, these things done in the name of weight loss, inevitably led to more weight (even if it was only a pound or two), more despair, less freedom, and, most importantly, less peace. This cycle was vicious, cruel, and frustrating … and often made me hate myself more.

Those things I did got the whole deal inside out.

I bought the false bill of goods that the promise of weight loss sold me—that being a certain weight or eating a certain way would automatically result in the things I wanted in my life appearing and staying … for good.

It wasn't weight loss or good nutrition I really wanted, it was the results they tantalizingly but deceivingly offered: Freedom and peace from obsessive thinking about food;

feeling good in my body; confidence; close connected relationships with those around me; an end to the shame I felt for being so concerned about something so, well, logically stupid; enjoying getting dressed; eating in social situations; taking pleasure (rather than sanctuary) in my food. Simply being okay with what I saw in the mirror and not thinking about food and weight and weight and food all … the … time.

I now have all those things I always wanted (way beyond grateful). I got them by practicing the steps I outline in this series of books, which details my journey to loving myself from the inside out.

This series takes an entirely new approach. You won't find seven easy steps to your perfect body. You won't be given the secret to an instantly brilliant life. I will, however, show you how I extricated myself from the hell that food was for me. Through my example, may you discover a path toward healing for yourself.

It's Got Nothing to Do With What You Eat

When you believe in yourself more than you believe in

food,

you will stop using food

as if it were your only chance at not falling apart.

~ Geneen Roth

I was shocked to discover that ninety-five percent of people who diet end up putting on more weight than they lose. Can you imagine a doctor prescribing a drug that results in ninety-five percent of those taking it worse off than not having taken it? Regardless of these grim statistics, doctors and nutritionists still prescribe diets (with the best of intentions, I imagine).

In 1950 a long-term, scientific study (The Ancel Keys Semi Starvation Study) was done on thirty-six men of the highest physical and psychological health to ascertain how few calories they needed to survive. In essence they were put on a strict, low-calorie diet. Along with a host of physical symptoms including declined metabolic rate, indications of accelerated ageing, depleted physical endurance, all thirty-six participants developed severe food obsession and, get this, distorted body image. You read that right. These perfectly healthy males with no prior food issues ended up not only stealing food out of rubbish bins, bingeing uncontrollably, obsessively dieting (then regaining more weight than they started with) - they became obsessed with getting thin, staying slim, reading dieting books and hating their bodies. Going back to how they used to eat and how they used to think about themselves was a difficult, long winded task and for a few of them, impossible.

Reading that study, I was compelled to share my approach to having a body I love. Tinkering around with food and exercise doesn't carry the day; it only deepens frustration, adds weight, and leads right to the gates of hopelessness and powerlessness.

If you use food to remove yourself from the stress of the world, or to quiet down thoughts that steal your peace and drive you mad, this series of books is for you.

Begin now to believe in yourself more than you believe in food. It is possible. Let me show you how.

My Story

The women I love and admire for their strength and grace did not get that way because shit worked out. They got that way because shit went wrong and they handled it.

They handled it in a thousand different ways, on a thousand different days, but they handled it.

Those women are my superheroes.

~ Elizabeth Gilbert

Life is no more worked out for me today than it was when I first started bingeing. In fact, my problems are bigger. But I no longer binge, purge, or spend fruitless hours stressing about the size of my thighs. I don't get lost down the bewildering rabbit hole called, 'I Ate Something "Bad" So I'm a Total Loser Who Has No Willpower.' Instead, I focus on leaving the world better than I find it, the quality of my relationships and the service I can be to others. These things are new and hard and on the far side of scary but… way more nourishing than any food I used to relentlessly shove in.

It's worth saying again—this series is not a set of easy

steps to magically make your life work out. The magic, indeed, if there is any, is that you will find strength to love and cherish yourself wherever you find yourself. That you will handle with grace whatever there is to handle in the rocky course of your life and food won't look like a good escape route anymore.

It has taken me years to switch from believing in, and wanting, a fairy-tale ending (where I'd sail into the sunset in my bikini-skinny body, all problems solved, nothing in my rosy world but ease and happiness) to living each day fully, knowing that today, this one we are experiencing right now with its mess of circumstances, is the only place I get to live a satisfying life.

When I discovered how to love myself, I found grace, strength, and self-worth. It is with compassion that I look back at my fourteen year-old self. I didn't know back then that choosing love would have saved me years of hell.

It was when I was fourteen that a family friend saw a photo and casually said (without, I'm sure, intent to harm), "Emma's not as thin anymore; she really is turning into an adult." That was it—self-hatred kicked in.

I looked at the photo and couldn't bear what I saw. Boiling, seething disgust and shame for my body rose up. Never before had I given my physical size the time of day. From then on, I couldn't stand it.

My self-hatred began with three thoughts: I am fat, I am

ugly, and I cannot live with this monstrosity of a body.

Something, I decided, must be done.

I locked myself in my room so lunch wouldn't tempt me. Hungry beyond sanity by dinner, I ate more than ever. And so it began. Going back again and again, trying to fill an endless hunger.

To compensate for over-eating I tried my hand, once more, at starvation. That lasted less than a day. I broke down and snuck food to my room and ate. And ate. And ate. The relief from the emptiness was so complete that I couldn't stop. It wasn't until I was past stuffed that a consciousness of what I had done dawned and with it a revolt so deep I could have launched a boat and sailed away.

The bingeing gave way to purging, and so it was for years and years.

Sometimes I'd go a week or more with relative sanity. Just keeping the binge at bay. I'd hardball these rough patches with the strongest of willpower; nails dug in, perpetually analyzing, controlling, strategizing, figuring out what was okay to eat and what wasn't. I'd make lists, commitments, promises to myself. Then, eventually, the desire to binge would overtake me and I'd cling to the hope that tomorrow would be different.

Tomorrow, sweet tomorrow. I'd be better. I'd be good. I'd

wake up and never touch sugar, or fat, or any kind of "bad" food again. Fantastically, I'd think, the desire to eat will be gone. I ate my way through a grocery store of food with the idea that tomorrow I would wake up sane and normal, slim, fit, and happy.

I chased ten pounds up and down the scale, gaining and losing it over and over and over and over again. I gave the number on the scale all sorts of uncalled-for power; to dictate my self worth; to say what kind of day I'd have; to preside over how I felt about … me.

By this time, twenty years in, I'd been in eating support groups, I'd read countless spiritual texts, I'd tried meditation and psychotherapy, I'd been to insightful and helpful self-development courses. All of which had a positive impact, but none of which offered the deep transformation I sought. Nothing, yet, had allowed me to embrace myself with the full unconditional love a mother instinctively has for her child; nothing allowed me to grasp my obsession by the hand and thank it, with deep gratitude. Nothing had shown me the amazing gift I had in my desperate hands but couldn't yet see. Nothing authorized me to love my obsession so fiercely I couldn't help but appreciate it for giving me a door into who I was. That, my friend, was yet to come.

True healing began in my late thirties in a small room in Los Angeles, where I moved for three months to paint. Disheartened with the same obsessive thinking that ricocheted around my tired mind, I finally had enough. It was my version of hitting bottom. I wasn't on the precipice of suicide, but I knew that if something didn't change, I'd never have the life I wanted. I would never be the person that the insistent nagging voice in my head kept urging me to be. Never. The battle would rage on until I died. A tired, old, worn out, never-ending war. I made a pact with myself. This is it. I will stop looking outside of myself to change how I feel within. I, from this day on, will stop trying to be different than I am. I will stop trying to escape my thoughts. I will stop fighting the binge. I will put down my sword. I will mimic the brave souls who love themselves, regardless of circumstances. I will be part of this energy called life. I will live with everything I have … even if I don't know what that means.

I promised myself I would find the gift in my obsession. I rose up to the clammy realization that the only way into myself was though the door of my dysfunctional eating. Until I was ready to journey, arms open toward my eating disorder and treat it as a portal to the part of me that is bigger than the content of my mind or the size of my bum, I would be stuck.

I decided to take on new practices. Not diets or gimmicks pretending to offer up a brand new identity, but practices that would establish a new pathway to being kind, loving, and accepting of … me.

If the obsession to eat calls, I thought, I will. Not just eat like I have been, but with lavish abandon and wholehearted enthusiasm. I will eat like Cheryl Strayed tells writers to write: like a motherfucker. I will bring humility, consistency, fun, fear, and every emotion I've squashed and run from, to the table. This will be my work. I will make food fully, abundantly available. No more tomorrows. No more chasing the elusive promise that managing my food (in whatever fashionable guise that might come in) will turn me into something I'm not. I will follow in the footsteps of my superheroes and mirror their relentless handling of shit.

I knew it was time to put the practice of "present moment allowing" to the test. The idea of simply allowing all of me to be exactly as it is and isn't. This notion couldn't have been more terrifying. Resisting is the cornerstone of addiction. Pulling out that block looked like an awfully dangerous thing to do.

I could see if my intention was to accept all as it is, I was going to have to give up the wishing, fantasizing, and desperate desiring for life to be different. No complaining about my lot. No bitching and moaning. That is a big pill to swallow. But that was my work.

I took on doing awkward uncomfortable things like talking to myself in the mirror. I made myself stand naked, face to face with the body I had hated so much for so long and vowed to care for her. I found the grace to apologize to every lump and bump. I set out to forgive and tried on allowing the hate I had nurtured up until then, to be okay. I told my body that while I couldn't promise that my automatic unconscious thoughts would never be negative again, I could promise that as soon as I noticed those septic thoughts, I would apologize, find contrition. In between bouts of almost uncontrollable tears, I told my body I would be vigilant about subjecting it to shaming. I vowed from then on to face each day with incessant, deep-seated self-love. There was much work to be done.

I gave up looking outside of myself for salvation. I had to stop thinking my problems were due to society, or my parents, my upbringing, my schooling, or the media. I was no longer going to abdicate responsibility for personal happiness to something nebulous and completely out of my hands. Anger, frustration, arguments—all of which were outside me—did nothing but keep me reaching for food, more and more food. It was time for me to understand where and when I was giving up and caving in. Not to the food, but to the incredible possibility I had to choose myself. To choose how I respond to what I face, at any given moment.

I wasn't sure I was up to any of the above, but I promised myself: I will learn. I will stand up for a life worth living. I will occupy a body I love. This is my chance at the life I always wanted. Bring me the key and I'll open the door.

The practices I outline in this book are a combination of those I took on before, and since, my time in Los Angeles. They are the foundation from which my healing grew.

I have purposely taken the practices that helped me know who I am and bundled them into Book One. Putting a stake in the ground and vowing to heal begins with the step called: I Will Understand 'Me.' This is the step from which all my healing rests on.

By understanding me, I'm not just talking about who I am as a mother and daughter and sister and lover and artist and woman and friend and what movies I like and what my deepest darkest secrets are and what embarrassing mistakes I've made and the shameful ones, too. I needed my understanding to stretch wider, without diminishing any of that. The practices I sought were ones that would open me up to who I was in the fuller scheme of the world. I wanted to know things like how the voice in my head related to the energy in my veins. How the body I walked around in connected to the environment I moved in.

I have skidded, tripped, danced, and deepened this mash of learnings and practices over the last ten years. They have formed the basis of my healing and (magically) have pried open my ability to see that the body I always wanted, a body I could love without reservation, was always there … patiently waiting to be seen.

My Promise to You

If you get the inside right, the outside will fall into place.

~ Eckhart Tolle

I'm not a trained doctor, therapist, psychologist, counsellor, life coach, scientist, spiritual advisor, or biochemist. But I do know what it's like to be obsessed with food and then, miraculously, what it's like to transcend the grip food can maintain. I have gone from every decision in my day being tainted with thoughts of eating, self-loathing and weight, to having space to build a creative career, be fully present with my family and at peace in social situations involving food. I don't weigh myself, plan what to eat, or not to eat. I don't beat myself up about eating more than I should. I don't despair at my own thoughts. I fit into the same clothes year in, year out. Food doesn't dominate me anymore. I have a burgeoning love for my body and a gratitude for the life I live. I took a journey that brought me home to myself. In the process, I experienced profound healing.

Can I promise you will heal, too? Yes and no. From a scientific point of view, I don't have a randomized, double-blind, placebo-controlled, peer-reviewed, experiment to back up my theories. In fact, I'm not sure I can call my experience theories. I only have my experience, what I have done and the results I got. I have read widely, enjoyed countless conversations, and formed solid opinions about what works ... for me. I have looked to the experiences of spiritual sages and scientists to try to understand why my practices have helped. That said, because this book is nonscientific, I suggest you take my experience as a starting point – a way to frame the beginning of your own healing. Take what I say, try it on, change it up, and make it work for you.

What I can say is if you look inward rather than outward to find freedom from obsessive thinking about, and eating of, food—you will. This is my promise to you. If you practice loving yourself from the inside first, you can fall madly, deeply in love with the outside.

Perhaps it's no coincidence this book is in your hands. Perhaps the time has come to put down self-hatred, self-doubt, frustration, and hopelessness . . . and pick up a much better way to live.

When it comes to having the body you want, the first book, Know Who You Are, will create a foundation for positive, long-lasting results. It has for me, and it has for others. To get access to this freedom and peace, simply read   on.

1: UNDERSTAND YOU

Mastering others is strength.
Mastering yourself is true power.

~ Lao Tzu

Healing, inventing, or transforming anything starts, as we know, with acknowledging there is a problem. We don't go to a doctor or therapist, or seek any kind of help until we admit something is wrong. Yet this step is far more than a simple admission (if you hadn't already admitted you had a problem, you'd hardly be reading this book, right?). It's stepping past admission and painting the landscape of you in intimate detail. It's understanding the unspoken tundra of your person. It's knowing the makeup of the soil and water needs, the sunshine quotients, the amazing array of plants that will grow, and recognizing the entire ecosystem your landscape supports. It's not about separating one part of you out (like the food you eat, the weight you want to lose, or the obsession you want gone) and focusing on that. What I'm getting at here is that while understanding yourself and acknowledging all that you are may sound like a simple step to take, in truth, it's not.

In my own healing, I've had to acknowledge my eating problem but also unravel everything else about myself. I had to look (and look again and again and again) at who I was and wasn't, and what I thought and felt and did and didn't have and wanted to be and dreams and loves and things I'd done to hurt others and things others had done to hurt me and what I was holding onto and held against people and what my feelings felt like and who and what I was scared of and how I fit into the mess of life around me. In other words, everything. No stone left unturned. I'd be lying to say it wasn't an unsettling, uneasy, messy process. It took me (and still takes me) to the edge of myself and further. I don't say this to frighten you. I say this to prepare you.

But let me say this, not all the work I did was terrifying, hard, and confronting.

Learning all the different aspects of "me" was an important part of knowing who I was. In doing so, I separated out the various "me"s of my being; my physical body from the voice in my head, and the awareness I had of those two things. And then, the very best bit, I got to see how all those pieces played their part in having the body I always wanted, by embracing the body I'd always had.

.

2: THE CREATIVE SOUP

The Creative Soup and You

In the beginning

There was neither existence nor nonexistence,

All this world was un-manifest energy

~ Hymn of creation, The Rig Veda

In this book, I draw a line in the sand between looking to fix myself from outside mechanisms, and turning my gaze inward to find healing. One of the most powerful instances in my journey, one that stands out as a step across that proverbial line, was that sublime moment of instant transformation, when I grasped how my individual being fit into the whole of nature. It was then that I first became aware of The Creative Soup, the place we all arise from.

I was listening to Deepak Chopra's silky, rumbly, accented voice while doing housework. His lecture talked about energy—specifically how it cannot be destroyed or created. It can only change form. I stopped in my tracks. I'd heard this in high school, but had never applied it to the energy flowing through my veins.

Energy can only change form!

The energy in me was not, could not have been, created from scratch. It was merely reorganized from somewhere else.

We are all part of a shared energy mass. I call this The Creative Soup. Creative because it is what we are created out of and Soup because everything you could possibly need is already in it.

My energy, the buzz I could feel as I moved about my house, existed before I was born and will go back there again when we die. Whoa, whoa, whoa. Something split open in me. I was part of something much bigger than the edges of my body. I was an ingredient in the Soup.

By the end of his lecture I knew:

- That every being on the planet is part of one huge mass of energy—we just arrive and do our thing in different forms; and

- This was trickier to grasp—the energy in me and around me has the potential to be anything and everything.

What if, what if, what if all this fight I'd had with my body was partly because I didn't understand the physics of it? How could I embrace the energy in me rather than fight it? How could I put this knowledge to use? How could I understand what was really going on at the level of this shared energy so I might work with it? Would doing so open a door to a body I love?

These were my dog-with-a-bone questions. They led me to the subatomic particles that create material existence to find the answers I was looking for.

What Science Tells Us

I think you'll find it's a bit more complicated than that.

~ Ben Goldacre

Armed with my questions, I entered the magnificent world of quantum physics—the place where construction and formation of matter is examined. As I delved into this fascinating arena of energy and particles, I realized the falsity of the information I'd had up until then about how nature works. Diet, exercise, and self-loathing as ways to change my body, when viewed through the lens of quantum physics, were ridiculous. Those things work to try and change something that isn't even real. It's akin to re-drawing a motorway on a map and wondering why the traffic problem hasn't changed. Any instance where we try to change the nature of our being in any kind of meaningful way from the outside in, I could finally see, was never going to work.

I mean, check this out:

- Energy and matter are the same thing. The way energy moves creates the illusion of solidity. Einstein realized this when he suggested his famous equation E=mc2, which essentially means that matter is made from energy that is moving extremely fast (twice the speed of light, to be precise). Once energy starts to move this fast, matter starts to appear solid, even though it's not really;

• Subatomic particles are more like energy waves that are in constant motion, and appear to come in and out of existence;

• These now-you-see-them, now-you-don't particles (or frequencies) are in a never-ending exchange game with the energy from other atoms (this microscopic environment is gravely unstable);

• Atoms are almost entirely made up of space. The relative spaciousness that subatomic waves of energy have to whizz around is the same relative spaciousness the planets have in our solar system. Can you even get your head around that? It's almost unimaginable.

All this adds up to three the-world-will-never-look-the-same-again things:

1) Atoms have no concrete boundaries or edges. The whizzing of their internal energy creates a sort of boundary-like illusion, which in reality isn't a boundary at all. This means the edges of myself that I see with my eyes are not real. Not even slightly.

2) Atoms are almost entirely made of space. Vast. Enormous. Almost inconceivable space. Which means I, too, am made up of this unimaginable space—nothing about me is solid.

3) Atoms are constantly changing. Down in this vast spaciousness, where energy is flying about, they are playing a never-ending game of swap out with energy from surrounding atoms. The energy in me is only here for a fleeting visit. It arrives, then hops away to be part of something else. My physical self isn't the same from moment to moment—wild!

I studied and studied and began to see why quantum physicists say the world we experience on a physical level is brilliant and beautiful but, still, a mighty deceptive illusion. The illusion? The perception that physical matter is solid and separate.

Nothing is what it seems.

This illusion, this complete misunderstanding of what is real and what is not, is at the heart of why so many suggestions about how to lose weight, get in shape, and eat right, fail from the outset. They work on the premise that we are solid and stable and separate and that we can somehow impose a set of limitations on our physical bodies from outside of us. But we can't. That's not how physics works.

The Illusion of Separateness

Reality is merely an illusion, albeit a very persistent one.

~ Einstein

Think about the sun for a moment. Conjure up an amazing sunset and sunrise; think about how the sun travels across the sky. Of course, in some respect, these are "real," but they are also a magnificent illusion. The setting and rising of the sun is only true from a certain, illusionary, vantage point.

In the same way that the sun travelling around the earth looks real from one point of view, but isn't really, the same mind-blowing, Alice-down-the-rabbit-hole experience of our physical separateness from the world around us is also deceptive.

Our separateness as individual human beings is true from the vantage point of our ordinary daily life and is extremely useful (my hands are writing this book), but that doesn't mean the illusion is real.

Believing it is real is where we get stuck. Very stuck. Of course we all enjoy sunsets. We talk about the sun being low in the sky, but by understanding that the earth travels around the sun, we also understand gravity, seasons, eclipses, and our place in the solar system, without having to make up myths and legends about why things are the way they are.

In the same way we have to pull back from the earth to see what is really going on with the sun, we, too, have to shift perspective, to see what is really going on with us. When we reconsider the whole, it allows us to hone in on those smallest of parts and the edges we think separate us from the world disappear. We become intimately part of everything.

We—you and I—become intimately part of everything.

But we must be individuals in some way, right? Or at least that became my question. Here I am, living my life and now you tell me my body isn't what I thought it was. It's not a solid, separate entity. It's a wiggle in The Creative Soup. But there is a me. There has to be. I'm aware of myself. I can see myself. I can hear my thoughts. I can make connections and feel love and write a book—this, surely, is me.

In asking these questions, I stumbled on what is individual about myself, It's not my physical body, but my awareness of it.

Our physical bodies may not be separate from the surrounding environment. But our awareness of ourselves is. Only you hold your awareness. Only I hold mine.

Once we begin to see ourselves from this truer perspective, all sorts of amazing power reveals itself.

The practices in this book are designed to help you connect with your awareness, which gives access to your power, and let go of the illusionary boundaries so many diets and exercise regimes are based on.

As I became aware of The Creative Soup and the illusion of separateness, I began to question the different "me"s inside of me, and how they fit together. I started to ask, how does the me that walks and talks and sits and runs and sleeps and eats, fit into, work with, and relate to, the me that is aware of all that, and—most importantly—the me that is the voice in my head that has opinions and beliefs and loves and hates and tells me I'm fat and feels ashamed and victorious and all those things (I call this voice The Resistance, but we will get to that soon).

These questions started a domino effect of learning.

The Importance of Awareness

Your ability to be conscious of yourself and your environment is unique to you. I walked around in a bubble of disruption for days when I learned my consciousness was the only thing about me … that was me. My consciousness is who I am. Yours is who you are.

Understanding this is what we New Zealanders would call—A Major.

To this point, Deepak Chopra says: You are not so much a human being that can have the experience of energy, but energy that is having the experience of being human. I had to read that over and over and over again. It wasn't until I understood the role of my consciousness that the light bulb went on. But then, bang, it all became clear.

Humans are the only creatures on earth that can be conscious of their consciousness. A horse, when it's cold, is cold. It doesn't know it's cold. It simply is cold. Or hungry. Once it isn't hungry, the hunger is gone. It isn't aware that it was hungry and then ate, it simply doesn't need to eat now.

We humans on the other hand have acute (and in my case, completely out of proportion) awareness of our physical body and the thoughts and sensations that arise from it. Where we get all mixed up is thinking our physical body is us.

As an aside, it was quantum physicists who cottoned onto the fact that everything is connected by energy, but it was philosophers who first realized human beings are the only animals who can be aware of that shared energy. Jean-Paul Sartre pondered Descartes's famous statement, "I think, therefore I am," and saw the fundamental error of it.

Eckhart Tolle, in The New Earth describes beautifully what Sartre discovered, "When you are aware of your thinking, the awareness is not part of the thinking. It is a different dimension of consciousness … If there was nothing but thought in you, you wouldn't even know you were thinking."

I knew I had woken up to my own awareness when I could distinguish the "me" that thinks from the "me" that is aware of my thoughts. I began to listen to the voice in my head like a radio station. I could pick out the role it plays in who I am, how I feel, the decisions I make, and the way I relate to myself. This awakening was transformative. It was one thing to know I am connected to The Creative Soup, it was a whole other thing to know the power of the voice in my head and that its job was to keep me from accessing my personal power. This voice was The Resistance.

.

3: THE RESISTANCE

The term "The Resistance" comes from Steven Pressfield. In the War of Art, he brilliantly digs into the voice in his head—the one that kept him from doing his work—and reveals it as the enemy of creativity. It's easy to see how the enemy of creativity relates to artists whose work is, by definition, creative. I'm extending the courtesy to everyone. Last I looked, all people are creative. I'm not saying that we all possess the talent to be a fine artist, but rather we all come from The Creative Soup. We all have a role in manifesting the stuff of our lives. To keep us reigned in, safe, and away from the danger of unleashing our creative force, we have … The Resistance.

In my early thirties, I read and read and read Deepak Chopra's Seven Spiritual Laws For Success and Eckhart Tolle's The Power Of Now. These guys call the internal human voice The Ego (to Pressfield's Resistance), but all three agree on its role and its power. The primary job of our internal voice is to distract us from our true selves, our conscious awareness. I devoured the teachings of these wise men, willing them to stick. In many ways they did. They certainly made a difference in my career. At the time, I made the leap to being a full-time artist. I learned to let go of the swill in my mind that told me I was a fraud, an impostor in a world I didn't belong, in grave danger of being caught by what Amanda Palmer (The Dresden Dolls) calls the Fraud Police and charged with being above my station and sentenced to eternal shame. That voice, I learned, was nothing more than mental noise pretending to be important. Because I knew this, I didn't get caught up in The Resistance when I set out to paint pictures for a living.

What I didn't do at the time, was connect the teachings in those books to the crazy food thoughts that were stuck on repeat in my head. Those thoughts remained like a special cause that I alone, due to my imperfections, had to bear.

I hadn't realized The Resistance toward my body had a malignant intention; to keep me safe … at all costs. The survival it was hell-bent on was a double-edged sword.

The Resistance kept me from burning my hands on hot stoves, crossing the road without looking and other such perils, but it also insisted everyone was judging me and it wasn't safe (not to mention good) to be me. The Resistance encouraged me to eat, to squash feelings, to fill the persistent emptiness, to escape the nagging sense I wasn't worthy of being alive, to hide myself from potential criticism.

The voice in my head that I'd done so much work on in my career, the one that told me I was useless and hopeless and a fraud and who was I to say I could be an artist, was the same voice that told me I was fat and ugly and no one loved me and if I could just be ten pounds slimmer all my problems would go away.

The thing I liked most about eating was that it shut The Resistance up. The rapturous peace from The Resistance was the reason for most binges. Having awareness of what The Resistance was out to achieve did two things: It gave me insight into why I liked to eat (to shut it up), and why it was so loud (to keep me safe).

Seeing The Resistance for what it is marked a massive turn in my healing. I was no longer at its mercy. I could step back and watch it. That small gorgeous step, right there, relieved me from a world of pain.

But, but, but … just because I was aware of it didn't mean it disappeared. Oh no—that would have been too easy. "I'm onto you, you big old resistance machine you," I'd think, and expect it to pack its bags and head south. But it didn't go like that. I'd hear something The Resistance was telling me and find myself desperately seeking solace with what went in my mouth to quiet down the relentless negativity. Ten bites in, I'd take a breath and observe, "Oh, shit, I've been hoodwinked." I had to learn to identify The Resistance and, harder still, step away.

This is what I know about The Resistance:

It is not who I am;

It is a bunch of crap that my mind uses to keep me safe;

It never goes away. It loses its power when I am aware of it, but it will always be there; and

Being aware of The Resistance is the work.

The tools, suggestions, and practices at the end of this book are based on what I did, and still do, to live beyond The Resistance and return to my awareness.

4: THE DIFFERENT ASPECTS OF "I"

Three "Me"s

Prying apart the real me from The Resistance left me enjoying a new understanding of who I was. I had gained ground in my healing. I didn't have to curtsey to a false master.

I began to connect the dots between:

- The Creative Soup (the energy we are all part of);

- The Resistance (the voice in our head that wants

us to be safe); and

- Who I am (the awareness of both of these things).

But there was more ground to cover. I saw there were three parts to myself, not just two. Over and above "The Observer me" (my ability to witness myself) and "Observations me" (the content of my mind), there is the "Observed me" (my physical body, actions, and thoughts).

At first, the distinction between these three was slippery to hold. I'd think I'd have the "me"s corralled, but then the horses would bolt. Now that I have them tamed, they help deepen my understanding of who I am.

Being The Observer

Rather than being your thoughts and emotions,

be the awareness behind them.

~ Eckhart Tolle

"The Observer" is the witness. It is consciousness. Awareness. Arising directly from The Creative Soup, it knows about connectedness, potentiality, love. It wants expansion. It sees potential and relentlessly nudges creativity to be fully expressed.

The Observer title makes consciousness active. It describes how to connect to The Creative Soup as well as what actions to take.

If you find yourself asking, "how do I witness myself," be The Observer. What are you observing? You. Your body, your thoughts, your feelings, your decisions, your actions, The Resistance.

When I am The Observer, two things happen:

- I step back and witness my life.

- I become present in the moment. It is literally impossible to be conscious, observe, and be aware at any other time than … now.

How do I know I am observing? I am aware of my thoughts, behaviors, emotions, and actions—like I am above myself looking at someone else. This way of being is new and different from my food-addicted life where the modus operandi was being pushed, shoved, and abused by my very own thoughts and emotions (The Resistance).

Being The Observer is a hard concept to get. So let's get concrete. See if you can be aware of the feeling in your hands. Be aware of the sensations. Are they hot, or cold? Can you feel what's going inside? Can you feel energy in them? Take a moment and close your eyes if you need to.

When you do this, you are observing yourself. You are bringing awareness to your hands.

Now, check your emotions. Can you be aware of an emotional sensation? Where is it sitting? How big is it? What color is it? How loud or dominant is it? You just witnessed emotion in your body.

See if you can catch The Resistance. See if you can witness a random unconscious thought.

That thought might be saying, "What thought?" That is the very one to witness. When you notice what you are thinking, you are The Observer.

I spent years thinking my thoughts were who I was. It's no wonder. This trick of light is common as dust. But still, absurd. Like thinking because a chair has a leg, it is a leg. Of course it has leg, but a chair isn't a leg. Nothing can be something it has. I have thoughts, but they are no more me than the leg is the chair. The "me" that knows I'm thinking is the real one. The thoughts that I think are "me" are the impostors. Bearing witness to my life is an elegant way to remind myself that I am not the parts of my life that I sometimes mistakenly believe I am.

This ability to witness comes right from The Creative Soup and arrives without judgment. The Observer has no opinions (they come from The Resistance); it is part of the energy of life. That means that when you are The Observer, you are not only observing yourself, you are also connected to the energy that connects everything.

When I first arrived at this beautiful (and for me intense) learning called "how to observe myself," I began to understand that my thoughts and feelings associated with food were close to unbearable. Please don't beat yourself up if you, too, get overwhelmed when attempting to be with thoughts and emotions associated with food. At first, I felt unhinged and had to go forward gently. The food and body-hate thinking that had dominated for years were not easy to witness, even when I knew, intellectually, those thoughts were only The Resistance.

The desire to relieve myself from this uncomfortable thinking was so intense I would cave. Then I'd feel like a loser for not being conscious enough to do what on paper seemed so simple—simply be with whatever there is to be with.

My work became observing those thoughts, too, the ones that were telling me I was doing The Observer thing wrong, that I would never get peace, that I'd never escape from my thoughts. When I saw this was just more Resistance rubbish, I saw the sneakiness of it; its desperation. That was big, that moment. I began to see the funny side. The extent to which The Resistance would go.

In the same way a broken bone can never be fixed so the break cannot be seen, the food addict lives with the stamp of her past. But there is beauty in this. A bone is either weakened or strengthened by its trauma. In the same way, we cannot undo breaks from the past, but we can take the broken bits and nurture them, accept them, build them into the canvas of our lives. These dings and scrapes are the very thing we take with us to others, to address the world with compassion and understanding. These bits swollen with life are the bits I now love the most. They are the bits that have opened my heart wider than I ever considered possible. They are the bits that drag my arse out of bed and make me hold out my hand to help someone else stumble past the block called impossible.

Witnessing the hate-filled internal voice will not automatically make it disappear. It doesn't send an evaporation ray to its heart, but it does put distance between you and it. It gives you the ability to send love to the wound and make that place in you stronger than it ever would have been without having lived through the injury.

I kept at it. Thought by thought, I did my best. I forgave myself for my slips, bumps, and jerky learning patterns. I was the weevil that wouldn't fall down. I committed to going back and back and back again until I could stay present to the powerful feelings and dark thoughts that drove me to eat. This presence, in the end, was my way through. The first time I sat and felt the full brunt of the storm The Resistance blew up inside me—urging me to lose myself in the pantry—was a powerful moment of healing. The thoughts and feelings eventually blew past and I was left peaceful and light. The next time those thoughts and feelings arose it was easier.

These days, the yearning to disappear into food doesn't visit nearly as often, but sometimes it still does. I notice. Curious. Like observing my children playing. "Hmmmm," I think. "Look at that. There's The Resistance, doing its thing." I'm in a continual dance of allowing, of observing, of giving my full attention. I practice being The Observer again and again and again and again. This is my work.

One more thing before we look at the "me" that is the observations: Self-awareness is the very thing that separates humans from other animals (opposing thumbs aside). It is why we say human beings are more evolved than others. More evolved doesn't mean better, more deserving, more entitled, worth more, it just means we have the ability to step away from ourselves and witness our thoughts, our actions, and our bodies. No other animal has the capacity to do this. My job is to practice using this gift and to use it well. That may not be the meaning of life, but it certainly adds to my sense of aliveness.

The Observations

Observation without evaluation

is the highest form of intelligence.

~ Jiddu Khrisnamurti

Observations me is tricky to get. That's because observations come through two paths:

1) From awareness—these thoughts don't judge or evaluate; they simply witness what is. These observations come from The Observer.

2) From The Resistance—these are highly reactive, judging, assessing, planning, scheming observations. They come with opinions and have at their heart a sense of analysis. Good versus bad. Me versus you. Us versus them. Right versus wrong.

If you are confused whether you are making an observation from The Creative Soup or from The Resistance, check in to see if the observation has an evaluation aspect to it. This is The Resistance.

Awareness is The Creative Soup observing its own creation. The observations from here are powerful, peaceful, detached.

The Observed

You don't have a soul.

You are a soul, you have a body.

~ Buddha

The me that I observe, like the me that makes observations, also seemed like the real me. My identity was intimately tied up with how I felt and what I looked like. I used to think I was unhappy, slightly pudgy, with fattish thighs and a bum that poked out. If you'd asked me, I would have said this is who I am.

I'd feel unhappy sensations (brought on by looking at the size of my thighs) and wallow around in a pit of despair. "Oh why am I so unhappy? What did I do to deserve this? What is the point of it all when I feel so bad all the time?"

I wasn't able to distinguish having emotion (oh, look, I have unhappiness in me) from the thought I am unhappy.

The Resistance loves this negative drama and body hatred because it distracts so well from creativity. It romances us down the enticing tunnel of self-pity ... "I'm sooooo miserable, I can't possibly create what I want until I feel better, I'll never feel better with these legs—may as well eat something".

The possibility of doing anything magnificent or magical or planet-changing while focusing on unhappy feelings is zilch. Doing big things requires stepping outside of emotion and knowing it's not who you are. The Resistance, as we know, doesn't like awareness or collective power. It doesn't like creativity. It doesn't like new. It only likes safe.

When I listened to the ever-present desire to expand myself and make a difference instead of wallowing, I had to take action in the face of screaming fear and high-decibel internal criticism.

I couldn't have done any of it without understanding that I am not my:

- Physical body, including flesh, bone, sinew, and synapse; or

- My thoughts, emotions, and sensations (in the form of Resistance), and the thoughts and feelings that arise from those emotions and sensations.

All of the above are the observed self. Nothing more, nothing less.

When I believed that the size of my thighs (along with the emotions I felt) was who I was, I tried everything to get better thighs, thinking that once I did, life would get better. The thing that took me a long time to learn, was that the quality of my life had nothing to do with the size my legs. I know because I kept getting to that perfect size and was still filled with self-hatred, shame, and despair. I'd eat to get relief. I would get bigger and once again I'd think my size was the problem. Around and around that merry-go-round I'd go.

The very act of distinguishing the three "me"s, allowed me to back out of that self-pity tunnel and head down a much happier path.

5: YOUR POTENTIAL

The last port of call to make, in knowing who you are, is understanding potential. In the days before I knew my potential, I was missing a fundamental clue called: What I am capable of. When I unearthed this precious constituent, I started to get a sense of the infinite options available to me.

I'm not talking about how fast you can potentially run, or the talent you have to get somewhere, or any sort of end-game scenario. I'm not talking about highlighting a future goal (getting a degree, becoming a doctor, making the team, being ten pounds lighter) and saying that is my potential.

I'm talking about what you are capable of right now, in this moment, in every moment. This is your potential.

I, for example, don't have the ability to sing to a crowded stadium. I don't have talent for singing or an ear for tune. That said, I have the potential right now to practice singing and enlist a coach. I can visualize myself in front of the crowd, if I choose. I can take actions aligned with an end goal ... any end goal, no matter how crazy or seemingly unattainable. This is what Mohammad Ali meant when he said:

Impossible is just a big word thrown around by small men

who would rather live in the world they've been given

than the power they have to change it.

Impossible is not a fact it's opinion.

Impossible is not a declaration it's a dare.

Impossible is potential.

Impossible is temporary.

In other words, you have the potential for anything. There is not an end goal that you cannot put a stake in the ground for and say, I'm working toward that. That is the direction I'm moving in today.

Does that mean you can achieve any end goal? No. But that's not the point. If you don't start something because you already believe you can't achieve it, you miss out on how close you may be able to get. You miss out on exploring your potential in this moment.

The question becomes, what do you want to achieve that you believe you can't? What are you giving up on before you even start? I don't actually want to sing to a crowed stadium. But I do want to enjoy getting dressed and take pleasure in my food and have crazy mad love for my body. I want to stay the same size season in, season out. I want to be fearless and open and alive. I want to write books that make the world better for people locked into hideous relationships with food. I want to write books that make the world better. Full stop. I want people to flourish. The beauty is—I can step strongly, or trembling, fast or slow, with abandon or precision toward all of that. Or not. My choice. My potential. Yours, too.

Seeing the difference between a choice to be on a path toward something and saying that thing is impossible is the difference between understanding your potential and falling into the trap of The Resistance.

The Resistance doesn't like the idea of potential. It prefers the notion of impossible and will try to convince you of it, every time.

The beauty of knowing I have the potential for everything, including the body I want, adds another string to my watch-The-Resistance-rather-than-listen-to-it bow.

Potentiality is a strong antidote to resistance. Where your potential comes from is important to understand. Let's go back to the Creative Soup and look at the origins of potentiality.

Your Potential and Nature

It is one thing to know The Creative Soup is where everything comes from. It's another to understand how The Creative Soup manifests what it does. This story points to Mother Nature and the way she operates. Her operating manual, if there were such a thing, would have "The Way of Potentiality" as chapter one.

When the door to my own potential opened, I wrote down everything I wanted. The list was long and included things like a body I loved and to eat with respect, ease, and open-hearted enthusiasm. I added feeling gratitude for my past experiences and using my experiences to help others heal. The desires on this list became the potential I stepped into each day.

As my new relationship to potential blossomed, a strange thing happened —the diets and exercise routines that I used to think would offer me the life I wanted, became the very things that started to arise from the internal changes I was making. As I got to know myself better and aligned my actions with potential, I naturally started to desire food that made my body feel good. I was motivated to exercise for the sake of it.

It would be a mistake, while reading this, to think that understanding the way nature works is an instant ticket to a blissful life. Understanding potentiality was nothing short of life-changing, but it didn't mean I never had to deal with my old ways again. I came to that more slowly. I'd gain ground, then fumble and slip. My old ways of being would creep in, and I'd have to reacquaint myself with what I'd learned.

How to Keep Potentiality Alive

Having awareness of potentiality gave me the courage to rekindle my desires. It allowed me to be okay working toward things I had no idea how to achieve. It stopped me from asking if what I wanted was possible and, instead, turned my head 360 degrees to ask what I could do to get myself one step closer to what I did want.

But I needed a way to make all I had learned about myself tangible on a day-to-day basis. Meditation is that way. Meditation gave me the physical experience of being connected to The Creative Soup, and reminded me that in it, exists the potentiality for everything. It put me in the witness box of my own life. Meditation dished up a daily serving of reality, allowing me to forget the illusion of separateness and continue to approach what I wanted for my life from the inside out.

Here is a taste of what I mean when I say meditation. As you read these words, see if you can be aware of the energy in your feet. If you can't, don't worry. Stop reading and take a moment to feel the energy with your eyes closed. The energy may be warm and lightly pulsing. Or quiet and faint. If you have been doing this for a while, see how much of your body you can sense while continuing to read. Can you feel your hands and toes? Can you feel the entire energy field of your body?

Notice you have to be alert. Your awareness must be tuned in. As you do the exercise and bring your attention to the energy inside you, you go more deeply into the present. Your mind activity subsides (even if it's for just a moment). There is nothing but silence and your awareness of The Creative Soup in you. This is meditation.

Meditation has been touted as one of the most powerful spiritual practices a human can do. While I agree, I have a unique perspective on how to practice it.

6: MEDITATION

The way I meditate has morphed over the years from being time-bound, to a present-in-moment practice.

When I first started, I set aside the same period of time each day to practice. I'd do twenty minutes in the morning and around ten minutes in the evening because, well, that approach was suggested. I was following the common advice. It wasn't a bad thing. It just didn't quite work in terms of connecting me to my awareness.

My meditation in those days became more about the time I was doing it than the quality of the practice. I'm not discounting the power of routine. Routines solidify habits and act as reminders to practice. The mistake I made was to think the routine itself was important, not the quality of the meditation.

When I practice true mediation, it doesn't matter if it lasts one second or one hour. I can only be aware now in this moment. One moment of full alert awareness is just as powerful as twenty minutes. One moment is certainly more powerful than twenty minutes of distracted shifting around on a cushion travelling to the past and future.

The funny thing is, when I used to practice time-bound meditation, time dragged and the practice felt burdensome and wasteful. Now that I simply go fully into my awareness, time slips away and I instinctively want to bring that practice to all parts of my life.

My current practice is not divided into neat chunks of life when I'm not meditating or I am meditating; it is more like, either I am fully present to what I am doing, or I am not. I can always bring my presence to a situation. I can always observe The Resistance, my body, and my actions. I can always practice more.

As my mediation practice evolves, I've found the following provide excellent access.

1) Spending time in nature.

2) Listening to silence.

3) Being alert to all my senses.

Spending Time in Nature

I have long enjoyed strong kinship to the natural world. The beauty and magnificence of nature has dished up countless stop-me-in-my-tracks experiences. The sense of infinite grandeur when standing on the top of a mountain looking at the ranges falling into incrementally faded triangles, or seeing a sunset festooned with color and heat and then, achingly, fade out, brings tentacles of energy spiking up my back, opens up crystalline awareness and leave me in love with life. All else, but a pulsing vitality and the view in front of me, cease to exist.

Without knowing it, being in nature and soaking up these moments of reverence were my first experiences of meditation. For just a moment, I would be so fully there, so alive, that my thoughts stopped. I sought these experiences out without being able to say exactly why. I imagined it had something to do with beauty, or the feeling of insignificance and infinity at the same time. In truth, it was the moment of being singular with everything, without having to consciously bring it about. The bliss of my thoughts dropping away, and my body, for that second, being okay precisely how it was.

I'd exit those moments full. Satisfied and solid with peace. Those two feelings were so rare in my world.

Spending time in nature is one of my favorite meditation practices. It can be as simple as feeling the grass under my feet and giving attention to air filling my lungs. It can be as soothing as standing on the shore and feeling the lap and pull of waves on my feet, watching the water with the attention of a lion watching her prey. Or, as fleeting as looking at trees swaying in the wind. The quick glance snaps me to, stopping internal chatter and allowing me to be present. It can be as uncomfortable as feeling the cut and slice of an icy breeze on my cheeks. Letting the sensation be felt in its entirety. Being aware of my body's guard against the brutal elements. Giving myself the gift of allowing, instead of fighting. In these intense times, I can fully engage with the way my body responds. The cower of my neck. The brace of my eyelids. The rush of my feet.

I can spend a morning hiking hard and fast up steep treacherous terrain, feeling my breath hurt and my muscles strain as my feet connect to the rocks, sand and tundra. Seeing the views as they appear and disappear in and out of sight as I move fast and intentionally.

I can sit quietly beneath a tree. Breathing and listening. Seeing the tree for what it is.

These are the ways I seek out nature.

These are the ways nature invites me to become an extension of the energy that manifest it. Part of The Creative Soup. Every potentiality open to me, at all times.

Listening to Silence

First thing in the morning before I get out of bed, and again when I sit down shortly after rising to write, I listen with all my attention until the vast, silent space where all possibility comes from sweeps into my awareness, like a dam releasing its river. It fills me completely. As this happens the edge of my body gives way (figuratively) and I become tuned into the space around me. I can sense this space both inside and outside of my physical body. As if my physical body becomes irrelevant and I experience space instead of matter. I am witness, indeed, to the creative energy that connects us all. It has a beautiful simplicity to it.

That said, listening to silence has been one of the hardest things I've ever learned.

The first time I heard the ever-pervasive silence (having intellectually understood the concept for years) was surreal yet profound; easy yet fleeting; quiet yet overawing. I was walking down a busy street having helped a friend at a trade show all day. I had talked nonstop with customers inside a huge windowless showroom from the moment the doors opened at 9am until they closed at 7pm. Totally beat and completely relieved to be outside enjoying fresh air, walking away after a satisfying, exhausting day. Without consciously choosing to, I became curious about the street

I was on—in particular the trees that lined the road and the light that danced on the leaves as they caught the breeze. As I watched, a silence expanded out beyond them, enveloping everything, absolutely everything, just fleetingly.

I was awestruck.

For the rest of my two-hour journey home, I tried to catch that silence again. Sometimes fleetingly I would, and then just as fast it would disappear. Two hours of trains, ferries, and buses slipped by as I focused on catching that massive silent space.

These days, two years later, I can hear the silence, at will, anytime. That doesn't mean I do hear it all the time. I get distracted by my thoughts and by what's happening around me, but I can always find it. I can always expand into the spaciousness.

To find that space, I focus on my breath and listen with all my awareness. The intention to go beyond what my ears can hear. I soften my gaze and imagine I can see beyond what I can see; the space between the atoms.

In those beautiful, graceful moments, everything but wonder fades away. For that moment, I am okay. I don't have an eating disorder, or a body I hate, or a problem to solve, or anywhere to go, or anything to achieve, or a fear to overcome, or an issue to deal with. I have nothing but the wonder and peace of the world around me, in me, waiting for the manifestation of the next moment.

These moments are gold. They are the ones where healing sets up camp and does its work. They are the instances that overshadow the grip of self-hatred and bring aliveness to the table. They are the spaces where love shines her bright torch and darkness is driven out.

Being Alert with All My Senses

The third way I practice connecting to The Creative Soup is to be alert with all my senses and feel the energy in me. I might lie down and feel the energy in my body or give attention to my hands as I'm walking.

As often as I can, I feel energy buzzing in my fingers, toes, and whole body. In the car. At the dinner table just before I eat.

I sometimes listen, not just to the silent space, but … to everything. The small clip of a coffee cup hitting the table. The happy pad of small feet running down our hallway in the morning. The wind. The rain. The shift and sway of fabrics as I walk.

I feel what my emotions are doing. Where they reside in my body. The quality of their urgency. The size, pitch, and insistence of their call.

I used to get battered by the onslaught of intense emotion. The self-hatred I had on replay in my brain was, I learned, accompanied by a mass of empty loneliness balled up in my gut. Black, dense and loud. It would sit there overtaking my day. Rather than try to escape that emotion, I've come to notice it. Be with it. Allow it. It cannot be filled up, that black hole. Ever. It cannot be escaped. Every time I eat to fill it, it comes back again, stronger. The only way through is directly in. Just being. Just loving. Just, just…

I practice observing all emotions that stop by and park up, or swing through fleetingly. There they are. There it is. Welcome. Can I help? Do you have a purpose? (Usually not.) Are you an old-timer? Have you been around before? Have I been trying to survive you for a while? Then you, little one, are even more welcome. You can have special attention. Wait, I sometimes suggest, until I can sit still and be with you. I always keep that promise. I always give my feelings the space and attention they need. It's when their time in the light is had, that they go. They shrivel up— their offering complete.

Nothing less and nothing more is needed. I don't need to analyze where they come from. The key is just … simply … being.

I consciously taste my food. Having spent years shoving food in, fast as I could, while distracting myself with TV, magazines, or a movie … I now pay attention. Do I like these flavors? What is the texture? How does this food sit in my stomach? What happens in my mind when I eat this food? Do I like these smells? Do I like the taste? Am I getting full? What kind of thoughts are swilling around when I eat this?

I pay attention with my eyes. I notice colors and people and look with purpose at the world around me. I take everything in so I'm left knowing … I really am here. When I pay enough attention, I become part of my surroundings. Because I know I am exchanging energy with my environment, I make a point of being aware of what I am exchanging with. If I don't like my surroundings, I limit my time there.

Sometimes, just for fun, I do a quick run through all my senses. Smell? Check. Visual? Check. Feel (including internal and external)? Check. Taste? Check. Sounds? Check.

This simple run-through is a way to connect to that which is bigger than me. Being aware of my senses helps me feel fully alive. It connects me to The Creative Soup. It grounds and straightens me out. It opens the gate to life.

.

7: PERSONAL INVENTORY

The last job in knowing who you are is to take an inventory of your life. Write the story, build the picture of your identity or ego, and examine all there is to see.

I did this exercise by writing down everything I thought, felt, had done, loved, hated, wanted to change, riled against, felt ashamed about, was embarrassed for or regretted, and also what my roles, jobs, etc. are. By being scrupulous in the endeavor I learned much about who I thought I was. The story of me contained page after page of stuff I had kept secret, unexamined, and tucked away for most of my life. There it was, alongside the stuff I'd discuss freely and frequently.

This pouring out did an amazing thing — it helped me see

that this collection of experiences, thoughts, feelings, happenings, fears, loves, and regrets does not define me. It was piles of anecdotes I mistook for me, but could stand aside and look at. I could love or hate the collection. I could examine it. I could make choices about it. I could feel the emotional charge of the content and then watch that charge go. I could release myself from it. Some of it happened in the past, that time had gone. Some of it was hopes for the future, but that had yet to come. I was free to soar above and beyond this series of words I had used to create an identity that had little to do with the reality of who I am.

It helped. It scrubbed a layer of hopelessness right off.

As a word of caution: I first took this step of inventorying myself, in the days before I had understood who I really was. That time, instead of a revelation, it sent me into a whirlpool of loneliness. It did nothing but make me focus on what was wrong with me. I didn't see, as I poured out the detail of myself, that the character developing on the pages did not reflect who I really was.

If you find yourself feeling worse after doing this exercise, go easy. Use the unease as a sign that you still believe the plot of your life is who you are. Revisit the ideas in this book and start again.

The second time I did this inventory, I had a completely different experience. With clear knowledge of who I really am, instead of being depressing, my sorrows were fascinating, dreams invigorating, shameful experiences one step removed.

It was nothing short of cathartic.

As I filled in this snapshot of who I thought I was, The Resistance quieted down. I understood with a clarity I hadn't had before as I wrote and wrote and cried and laughed and wrestled, that I was so much more than I had lead myself to believe. I could clearly see the stuff The Resistance had convinced me was important but, in truth, wasn't.

This was another powerful antidote to The Resistance.

In her "Dear Sugar" column, Cheryl Strayed wrote to a courageous man who had done much work on himself and, yet, found himself still wondering why he wasn't fixed.

"That it feels different here on this shore than you thought it would does not negate the enormity of the distance you traversed and the strength it took you to do it."

Try to let go of what your life will look like on the other side of this practice. Life will still come at you. That doesn't mean it's not worth doing. It does mean you still have your past, your parents, the same community you always had. You will always take that with you. But you are also strong and courageous and you have the power to see The Resistance for what it is. You have taken ground.

And so we come to courage. Taking this step to understand yourself requires standing up and taking responsibility for your life. It is saying goodbye to the idea of someone else fixing you. It is acknowledging that it's up to you to do the work. That's powerful, plucky, and an act of radical self-love. Which is a momentous and beautiful thing. You are making the world a better place. You are making your life a better one to live.

The Inventory

Get a notebook and pen and on the cover, write your name. On the inside, write: Everything I know about the 'me' I think I am.

You could create a digital document if you prefer, but I recommend writing by hand, as it elicits information in a way that typing won't.

Commit a block of time each day for a week. At least half an hour. That is a big call, I know. If you can't do half an hour, do what you can. Grab five minutes, or one. Don't stop from starting. Do some every day. Keep going.

Begin answering the following questions. As you do, remember there is no certain number of questions to get through each day, or week. Each of us will have longer or shorter answers for the same question, as we all carry different stories. Write until the answer is enough for you.

Trust the process. You'll know when it's time to move on to the next question. Don't try and answer "properly" or figure out why these questions are important. The important thing is to answer with whatever arises. Take the time you need for each question. There are no right or wrong answers.

This is an activity where it's important to just keep writing. It may help to write for defined periods of time (between 5 and 7 minutes), but keep writing. If you are stuck, write "don't know" or "what next" to keep you writing until the next thought arrives.

Censoring happens when we try to make our writing "pretty", or edit as we go—but the point is to write what is there.

Answer each and every question even if you don't know the answer (start by writing, "I don't know, but if I took a guess it would be …"). Go back over your answers and write more if you need to. How will you know if you need to? Because you won't ask yourself, "have I answered that completely?" You will know. If you are wondering, keep writing.

Take a different colored pen and circle the answers where you describe times you were abused sexually or physically. Do you feel peaceful about those situations? Have you ever told anyone? If you feel anything less than complete about them, now is the time to take action. (Google help in your area, check out references, look for local helplines.)

Now is the time to talk to a trained professional (In your search, be sure to check out Dr. Suzanne Gleb). Healing from food and body obsession is not going to start without letting go of the shame and fear that lingers from abuse. This is your work. It is the step to take. It might be the scariest, but it will be the best.

If you can't bring yourself to tell anyone about abuse that has happened, keep writing until you can. Take the step called 'I will allow myself to want to tell someone.' We cannot un-do abuse, but keeping it secret gives The Resistance license to keep you small and scared. Sharing it will put it in the past. When it's behind you, you don't have to keep re-feeling the fear again and again. You can let the trauma go. You and your body can heal, recover, and move on. Like the broken bone I described earlier, you will carry the scar, but you may be the stronger for it.

When you have finished answering your questions (this might take a week; it might take a year), I would suggest burning your book. If this causes a strong reaction in you, don't force yourself. I loved the ritual of burning because it acted as reminder that there was nothing in my story that is really me. All those stories were gone, literally and figuratively.

You story is your experiences; it has nothing to do with what's happening right here, right now. It has nothing to do with The Creative Soup, your ability to witness yourself, or the potential in you to take any step. You may want to keep your writing to revisit. You may want to burn it. If so, do it now.

Questions:

- How much do I weigh?

- How often do I weigh myself?

- What am I waiting for in life?

- What is my biggest secret?

- What is my biggest fear?

- What is my biggest dream that I don't think I'll ever achieve?

- What have I given up on?

- What don't I like about my life?

- What do I like best about my life?

- What parts of my body do I like the least?

- What parts of my body do I like the best?

- What do I eat that I think I shouldn't?

- What do I eat only because I think I should?

- What am I good at?

- What have I been doing over and over again and expecting to get a different result?

- What patterns exist in my eating?

- How old was I when I started obsessing about my eating? What happened at or around that time?

- What did my parents tell me about food?

- What did other children say about my body or my eating habits?

- What comments have I received about my body or my eating (over the course of my life) and by whom?

- What sexual abuse have I experienced? Who was involved? How old was I? Where was I? What happened? Who knows about it? What was the result? How did I feel at the time? How do I feel about it now?

- What physical abuse have I experienced? Who was involved? How old was I? Where was I? What happened? Who knows about it? What was the result? How did I feel at the time? How do I feel about it now?

- How many diets have I been on?

- What thoughts do I have about my body?

- Who has hurt me?

- What am I most afraid of?

- Who has done unforgivable things?

- Who has wronged me?

- What have I done that I cannot forgive myself for?

- How have I wronged others?

- Who have I not forgiven? Who cannot be forgiven?

- What are the persistent thoughts I have about my body and food?

- How much binging and purging did I do? When did it start? When did it stop (if it has stopped)?

- What do I feel ashamed of?

- What would I like to change about myself?

- How much money do I make? Do I earn more than I spend? How do I feel about money? Is my financial situation stressful or liberating?

- What do I do for work? Do I like my work?

- What roles do I have in my life? Which ones bring me the most pleasure? Which ones bring me the most grief?

- What is my relationship like with my family? What were the eating patterns of my family?

- What is the scariest thing that ever happened to me? What happened after that? How did I deal with it?

- What do I feel unworthy of? What do I feel entitled to that I don't currently have?

- How do I feel about my parents? What was/is my relationship with them like? What do I blame them for?

8: TOOLKIT

Practices to Understand Who You Are

Today I commit to the following practices:

1)   I will listen to silence as often as possible. I will practice listening to the vast space we all come from.

2)   I will make a list of three activities I do on a daily basis and bring my awareness to them. I will bring my attention to them like a cat watches a mouse hole. Alert, aware, and intensely focused in the moment.

3)   I will practice using all my senses. I will notice what is going on internally. I will begin to understand what fear, love, irritation, humility, and compassion all feel like; where they reside in my body, the intensity of them, what happens to my thinking when I feel those things. I will become like an archaeologist curiously uncovering an ancient city; I will learn every nook and cranny of my sensual self.

4)   I will feel the internal energy in my body on a daily basis. I commit to feeling the energy at certain points during the day—like when I first sit at my desk, or just before I get up in the morning, or just as I go to bed at night, or just before I turn on the television, or before I turn on the ignition in my car, I will feel that energy as deeply and acutely as possible.

5)   I will spend time in nature every day. Whether it is looking at a plant, swimming in the sea, hiking up a trail, or noticing a flower, I will notice the power of nature and practice seeing it as myself.

6)   I will continue to read books that connect me to awareness. I will continue to educate myself in the area of energy, and I will deliberately connect to that energy.

7)   I will take a regular inventory of myself. Once every year or so, I will look at what I've started believing is me and examine what I can let go of. I'll answer the questions in the Tool Kit. I'll reignite my creative desires and work toward them.

Key Concepts

The Creative Soup: The energy in us that can be found in everything.

The Resistance: The inner voice that wants to keep you safe at all costs.

Potentiality: The potential that exists in each moment.

The Illusion of Separateness: The boundaries of who it looks like we are is an illusion. We are not separate individuals at all, we are all part of The Creative Soup.

The three "me"s:

- **The Observer**—Awareness that arises directly from The Creative Soup. It knows about connectedness, potentiality, love. It wants expansion. It sees potential and relentlessly nudges creativity to be fully expressed.

- **The Observed**—The physical body: Flesh, bone, sinew, and synapses; thoughts, emotions, and sensations (in the form of The Resistance); and the thoughts and feelings that arise from those emotions and sensations.

- The Observations—Arriving one of two ways: From a place of awareness, these thoughts don't judge or evaluate; they simply witness what is. These observations come from The Observer. Or, from The Resistance—these are highly reactive, judging, assessing, planning, scheming observations. They come with opinions and have a sense of analysis at their heart. Good versus bad. Me versus you. Us versus them. Right versus wrong.

Meditation: The moment we become the witnessing presence to ourselves.

9: 'TIL WE MEET AGAIN

I started this book saying that I was nineteen when I told my parents I was bulimic. Twenty-six years later, I look back at that sad, scared teenager and have nothing but compassion. She lived a life so uncomfortable that the choice to grow, learn and love proved an easy one to make. The work to follow through on that choice is a different story. It's been by far the hardest thing I've done, but the choice itself? A no-brainer.

I thank that young me on a daily basis. Today, I know that every binge, purge, every hole of blackness she inched her way though, helped create who I am today. And if that is what it took to have what I have now, I'd choose it all again. In a second.

Without the knee-deep shit I waded through, would I have

bothered understanding quantum physics, The Creative Soup, or recognized the illusion of separateness? Would I have felt the moment of bliss where silence stitched itself into the seam of my soul? Would I have fought to understand the three different "me"s and how each of them impacts my life? Would I have paid such close attention to what potential is? Would I have wrestled with the words in this book so that you, beautiful one, can let go of the false premise that changing yourself from the outside will change you on the inside? Would I have issued this invitation to a journey toward who you really are and where you will find bountiful power?

I can't imagine why I would have.

As the words have laid themselves, one by one, into the manuscript of this book, I have retraced the steps of my own journey.

I'm reminded of the gift that younger me left for the older me to open and enjoy and in the reminding, I'm grateful beyond words. I understand that the gift grows exponentially when offered to others. My hope is that it will water a seed of self-love in you and that your seed might soar toward the light, rooted in awareness.

The work in these pages takes grit, commitment, living out on the thin branches of life. Each step you take toward understanding yourself will help you know yourself in an entirely new way. You'll know what is real and what is a figment of The Resistance. You'll have the tools to step back and watch the boil of emotion and sensation and negative thoughts as they come and go from your body. You'll have clarity about the different aspects of yourself.

Best of all, I hope you no longer seek to find a better tomorrow in the food you eat today. You can leave the false promise of diets and weight management regimes behind. You can unveil the enormous potential of yourself and rethink what is possible for your body, the way you eat, and the relationship you have with food. The next book in the Love Your Body, Change Your Life series is called Radical Self-Acceptance. Now you know who you are, I want to take you on a journey of accepting every beautiful inch of yourself. I look forward to seeing you there.

Keep Informed and Help Others

If you would like to know when I publish new books, sign up for my readers group/updates at emmawright.co.nz.

If this book helped you, there are two ways you can share the gift.

First: Amazon reviews are invaluable. If this book made an impression, for better or worse, please leave a review.

Second: Recommend this book to friends who might like, value, or appreciate it. Word of mouth is the best kind of endorsement.

If you want to say hello, or have any questions, email me at emma@emmawright.co.nz.

To check out my blog and latest projects, go to emmawright.co.nz

Thank you. Thank you. Thank you.

X

ABOUT EMMA

When I was thirty-seven, I forgave myself for having an eating disorder and for being single and childless.

In that moment, I also found out who I was.

I knew right then that I (like you and everyone on the planet) have great personal power, but often fail to use it.

Self-love changed the course of my life, healed my wounds, empowered those around me, and transformed the world I live in.

It all depended on one thing: being ready to surrender.

I have devoted my life to understanding how human beings operate—and how we can more fully be ourselves.

There is always more to learn.

My Work and Career

I am the author of two books (so far). *Feel Good Friday: 40 Unexpected Ways To Feel Good About Your Life* and this one, the first book in the *Love Your Body, Change Your Life* series.

I have sold over five hundred paintings to clients all over the world.

I've been profiled in magazines and newspapers in four different countries.

I teach an online course called 28 Days of Goodness, designed to put some of the ideas in my books into practice.

I've been self-employed for over ten years.

I have been called "brilliant" and "wise" by some; "frivolous" and "unoriginal" by others.

It has been an eye-opening road.

It all started in front of a mirror, uttering the words, "Emma I forgive" ... and shedding a bucketful of tears.

Other Bits and Bobs

I was born in Auckland, New Zealand. I currently live on a small island off the coast of Auckland with my partner and our two young children. My favorite human is Sai Maa. My favorite poet is Rudyard Kipling. My favorite spiritual leader is Eckhart Tolle. At one point in my life, I was a brand consultant for a graphic design agency. I love sunsets, all kinds of books (from literary to spiritual, biography to business nonfiction), coffee, movies, fashion, writing postcards, swimming with my children, and, of course, any opportunity to write, converse, create, and grow.

Also? I am much happier since turning forty. Forgiveness is beautiful.

For now, I reckon that's all you need to know.

18065222R00058

Printed in Great Britain
by Amazon